CHILD OBESITY
AS A MONSTER

EMMANUEL OJEMEN

BACKGROUND

Childhood obesity and its associated health risk is on the increase around the globe. No country is exempted from this monster.

Overweight children are at risk of suffering psychosocial problems like, low self esteem, low self confidence, poor body image, symptoms of depression and health issues like type ii diabetes, high blood pressure, bone issues, etc.

There are a couple of factors that contributes to children becoming obese. Nutritional factor, Sedentary factor, choices, environment etc.

This book is not just going to talk or explain only the problems, but will spend more pages proffering solutions, which is the role of nutrition and physical activities in tackling this monster that has landed in the planet of our children's lives.

HOW TO READ THIS BOOK?

Check for definitions

Check for conversations

Check for sample sentences

CHAPTER 1

THE NATHANIEL EXPERIENCE

Times for school sports or plays are very important to children in the school. No child loves to have his or her play time taking away.

Fridays are usually general PE days at city primary school and it's also a time for some selected and special sports.

The school has four sports clubs that students can choose from. Taekwondo club, Swimming club, Table tennis club and Badminton club.

Nathaniel prefers the Swimming and Badminton clubs, but you can only choose one per session. Nathaniel happily chooses Swimming with the hope of learning how to swim before the end of the year.

On this very Friday, the swimming club members were all outside waiting for the school's shuttle bus to take them to the Swimming pool.

Did I mention his age and body weight?

Well, his name is Nathaniel, but he's called Nat for short. He is 9 years old, and he is in year 4, that's primary 4

Surprisingly he weighs 70kg already.

It all started from a remark his classmate made, the mate said, the swimming pool will get empty once Nat jumps into the pool. Meaning his body weight would splash all the water out of the pool and everyone roared in laughter. Nat immediately became weak and downcast.

Been obese has pushed Nat away from activities he used to enjoy and loved doing just because he gets bullied as a result of been obese

Ďèffìñìtìòñs

"Obesity": Having excessive body fat that increases the risk of health problems.

"Risk": Exposed or opened to danger

"Excessive": More than is necessary or required.

"He was drinking excessive amounts of soda"

Obesity usually comes from taking more calories than you burn either by exercise or your daily physical activities.

No child loves to experience what Nat experienced. Such experience can go a long way destroying a child's self esteem, self confidence and self worth.

Let's have a peep into Nat's life.

COACH: how are you Nat?

NAT: I am fine Coach.

COACH: I see that you haven't been participating in sports and physical plays of recent

NAT: yeah Coach. Am just tired of it all....

COACH: Tired of what now?

NAT: Classmates, when ever I walk around, they laugh at me and call me names, when I run, they joke with it, when I try to join in conversation, they call me names.

COACH: Really!!! Why would they do that? Do you have any quarrels or fight with them?

NAT: No coach, just because of my weight, and its seriously hitting on me. Incant do anything or move around in school without been bullied.

COACH: It's okay Nat, I will in conjunction with the school do something about it. I promise I will.

NAT: Thank you coach.

Ďèffïñìtìòñ

In conjunction: Means.... "together "

What Nat is going through in school is happening to a lot o children every where in the world. A lot of countries are doing all they can to control Child Obesityy and Obesity bullying.

I know the UK is particularly all out to tackle it and its associated consequences.

CHAPTER 2

HOW DID HE GET HERE?

There are contributary factors to children's Obesity, Nutritional influence, Sedentary influence, Environmental influence, Choices and so on.

Despite the various factors, choice seem to be the scapegoat. The reason for captioning CHOICE as a dominant factor or influence is the fact that it controls the final decision that was made or taken.

NUTRITION

The types of food we consume goes a long way determining how we look and weigh on the scale.

Within nutrition, there are classes of food.

1. Carbohydrates

2. Proteins

3. Minerals

4. Fats & Oils

5. Vitamins

6. Water

Let's do a little explaining of these classes of foods to Nathaniel.

CARBOHYDRATES

This food class are the ones that are very high in their starch content and provides the body with glucose, the main energy source the body needs to function.

Examples of carbohydrates foods are Potatoes, Rice, Vegetables, Quinoa, Cakes, pastries etc.

PROTEIN

This food class provides the amino acid the body requires and It helps build and repair cells and body tissues, including the skin, muscle, etc.

Examples of food rich in proteins are Eggs, Lean chicken breast, Lean pork, Fish, Beef, Lentils etc.

MINERALS

Minerals are the elements in foods that the body need to develop and function well.

Examples of minerals are calcium and iron mostly found in meat, cereals, fish, milk, fruit, vegetables and nuts.

FATS & OILS

Sometimes refer to as fatty acids and glycerol. They are the main components of our vegetable oils and fatty tissues in animals. Fat gives the body energy, protects the organs and supports cell growth.

Examples of food rich in fats and oils; Butter, Cheese, Avocado, Seeds, Nuts, Cooking oil etc

VITAMINS

Vitamins helps the body grow and work the way it should. There are 13 essential vitamins — vitamins A, C, D, E, K, and the B vitamins.

Examples of food rich in the various vitamins; Watermelons, whole grains, Avocado, Broccoli, Mushrooms, Strawberries, Citrus Fruits etc

WATER

A transparent, odorless, colourless, tasteless liquid, that keeps the body hydrated, skin supple, and maintain the fluid in the body.

16

Nutrition comes with various options of foods for Nathaniel to choose from, the final decision is also left to him and his parents. Their collective decision will determine if the door will be opened for this Monster to come in. Sadly, Nathaniel has the Monster standing in front of him already.

CHAPTER 3

SEDENTARY LIFESTYLE

Another contributary factor to becoming obese is lack of physical activities. Quite a number of children worldwide move around less these days. The pandemic did more damage in locking them further indoors. Children constantly eating and yet not having times to burn all that are stacked in their bodies. Children are now connected more to their gadgets that make them immobile for lengthy hours. Online learning, online mandatory schools, social distancing and eventually the fear of contracting the corona virus have all kept them behind bars.

ENVIRONMENTAL FACTOR

The environmental factor can be described from two angles, the physical environment and the social environment.

Physical environment relates to neighbourhood that the children live in. Firstly, majority of the children live in poor neighbourhood where there are no infrastructures for neighbourhood plays and sport, this in turn keep them away from playing. Some other neighbourhoods are crime infested and parents don't want to risk losing their children to death or injuries or even been arrested and jailed. Children spend more times indoors and consuming unhealthy foods.

Social entertainment just like the physical environment relates to the activities and management of these activities to the benefits of the children. When the children are not managed or controlled within the physical environment with a social approach, they can also come up with lots of defective behaviours that are learnt from these places.

CHOICES

The choice that you make as a child can go a long way determining if you will become obese or overweight. As parents also, we must make fantastic choices un-behalf of our children.

Ďèffìñìtìòñ

"Choice": an act of choosing between two or more possibilities or options

Sample sentences: "the choice between good and evil"

Choice is a strong determinant in the decisions we make, whether good or bad. Nathaniel's body weight and psychosocial problems are a product of the choice or choices he and the parents made. It is therefore very important to evaluate all the options we have before taking a decision.

Ďèffiñitiòñ

"Determinant": What affects the nature of outcomes

"Evaluate": To judge or calculate importance

"Psychosocial ": Relating to the influence of social factors on an individual's mind or behaviour.

CHAPTER 4

HELP

Let's dedicate chapter four to create help plan for Nathaniel.

What do you think Nathaniel needs to deal with this monster?

"Jaron"

First and foremost, I think Nathaniel needs to embrace the fact that he's the way he is. So let the school mate deal with that.

"Jorah"

In her own opinion, Princess Jorah believes Nathaniel should mind his own business and forget about whatever people say and make up his mind to enjoy playing out there.

"Blossom"

Nathaniel should start by eating healthier food and stop eating late dinners. He also encourages him to embrace exercises, like riding a bike. You know bike riding is very fun.

"John"

He should just accept his body the way it is now but with the plan to make it better in the nearest future by setting a major plan out.

His parents can help him out of this.

"Grace"

I think his case can be reported to the school to caution those other children body shaming him. People can commit suicide from these types of cases if not checked. The school should play a role here.

Ironically, the solutions to Nathaniel's problems are linked with the same contributary factors.

Firstly, Nathaniel and his parents should take a deeper look at his psychosocial life and deal with his insecurities like low self esteem, low self confidence, low self worth, poor body image and others.

Truth is, if you don't value yourself, how will people value you? If he doesn't believe in himself, who will believe in him? Its time for him to take the bull by the horn and wrestle with it.

(Picture of him wrestling with a monster here)

Another solution is the nutritional aspect. Nathaniel's dietary plan should be reviewed, and a new plan adopted for him.

There are other factors within nutrition that can help.

1. The type of food:

2. The frequency of eating:

3. The time he eats:

4. The quantity of food he eats:

The above four suggestions will help him to a large extent.

Children's diet should not be changed just because of what we feel as parents,

because children grow in unpredictable ways. It should only be done by a health care professional, using the child's height and weight relative to his previous growth history.

Physical Activities is another solution to solving this problem. Apart from food, type of food, frequency of eating and quantity, Nathaniel must get up from his butt's and hit the playground or field.

A coach should be hired to draw out a plan for him to follow daily because of the complexity of children's physical activities.

Children's levels of physical activity are highly variable and may be influenced by a multitude of factors including physiological, psychological, sociocultural and environmental determinants.

The prevention and management of child obesity is in our hands and as such let's join these same hands to defeat this monster.

Advisory

- Discourage children from eating their food and snacks in front of the TV. This makes them to eat without feeling full because the TV takes their attention away and they end up eating more.

- Make dinners early for overweight children. Late dinners contribute to the whole struggle.

- Make their dinner light but of quality meals.

- Reduce their screen times and days to weekends only. This will help them move around more and get active. Sedentary living contributes to been overweight

- Make outdoor plays compulsory for the whole family rather than just the overweight child. Group plays encourages them more than been alone in the activities

- Incorporate intentional exercises into their day. Make them use the stairs rather than the elevator, walk to near destinations with them.

- Make them a part of the planning of the grocery. Tell them the reason why somethings are not needed in the house and why some of them are a must

- Put them in charge of the process of implementation. Adopting the idea earlier than other members of the family will encourage him or her to take responsibilities

Ďèffìñìtìòñ

Contributary: "Playing a part of in bringing something about".

Grocery: "Items of food sold in a supermarket".

Sentence…. I bought groceries for the family

Compulsory: "Something that is a must"

Incorporate:

Intentional:

Implementation:

www.ingramcontent.com/pod-product-compliance
Lightning Source LLC
Chambersburg PA
CBHW050713250726

48662CB00002B/993